36 Beauty Secrets

Greatest Beauty Tips Of All Time

Ann Savage

ANTI-AGING SKINCARE SECRETS REVEALED

How to have your skin Beautiful In

The Next 10 Days

Your Free Gift

As a way of saying thanks for your purchase, I'm offering a free guide that's exclusive to my readers.

In this guide, you will learn how to turn any messy room in into a nice, clean, and tidy room, cleaning in only 3 hours. Your home will stay clean every day and you will never have to worry about unexpected guests walking into a dirty house again. You can download this free report by going here.

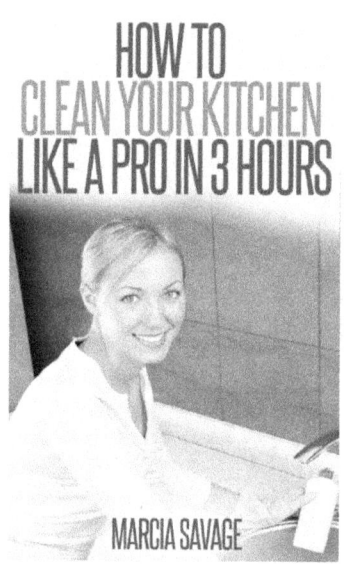

http://forms.aweber.com/form/76/315836976.htm

Table of Content:

Brown Sugar Facial Scrub

Cucumber Mask

Cucumber Lemon Mask

Cucumber Yogurt Mask

Lemon Honey Facial

Lemon Banana Facial

Lemon Egg White Facial

Lemon Skin Toner

Watermelon Skin Toner

Tomato Skin Toner

Rice Skin Toner

Rose Water Skin Toner

Witch Hazel Skin Toner

Green Tea Skin Toner

Lemon Oil Skin Toner

Tea Tree Oil Skin Toner

Rubbing Alcohol Skin Toner

Peppermint Tea Skin Toner

Egg White Yogurt Hair Conditioner

Honey Coconut Hair Conditioner

Honey Olive Oil Hair Conditioner

Honey Mayo Hair Conditioner

Coconut Milk Banana Hair Conditioner

Avocado Banana Hair Conditioner

Affordable Natural Skin Care

Hello, my name is Ann Savage and I would like to personally thank you for purchasing my book. I have added skin care recipes that have been in our family for over 100 years for you to test. Please leave your opinion about these recipes to help others.

I would also like for you to email me your recipes for me to try, giving me permission to add them in my upcoming books for other people to try. I will list your name as the provider of the recipes and add you to my newsletter to be notified when my new books are release. Email me at:

bsavage50@windstream.net

Warning, Warming, Warming

Sample all recipes before using. I am not a doctor or a dermatologist and I cannot give any medical advice. This are skincare products that have worked successfully for years for other people I know. Please test all products before using them to ensure you're not allergic to the substances within the product.

Here some of the produces listed in my recipes and the benefits for your skin:

Apple Cider Vinegar will help restore your skin's natural pH. balance and is a great cure for acne.

Avocado is a moisturizer and calms skin irritation.

Bananas are a great moisturizer for dry skin.

Brown Sugar is good for exfoliation.

Carrot contains antioxidants that have age fighting properties.

Cucumber can act as a natural astringent. It helps to reduce oiliness and tighten pores. It can also improve texture and help reduce dark spots.

Egg Whites are great for tightening your skin and shrinking pores

Honey is great for people with dry skin because it's moisturizing.

Milk helps you have soft skin. If you have rough skin, milk will help keep your skin soft.

Rice contains vitamins B, K, and E, which are anti-aging remedies because it helps smooth out lines and wrinkles.

Rosewater is great for normal to dry skin. You can purchase rosewater at most health stores.

Tomato has vitamin A and C, which removes blackheads and acne, helps with oily skin, and tightens the skin.

Witch hazel is a gentle astringent that's great for normal to oily skin.

Apple Carrot Facial

Ingredients:

1 Tbsp. Apple

1 Tbsp. Carrot

1 Tbsp. Cucumber

Step One: Cut the apple, cucumber, and carrot in half and grate into a bowl. Squeeze the mixture to remove all the moisture and mix together.

Step Two: It's hard to keep this solution on your skin so take 3 paper towels, put one on top of the other, and cut holes for your eyes. Wet it and pour the mixture on the paper towel and place the paper towel over your face. Leave solution on for 25 minutes and wash your face with warm water.

Apple Honey Facial

Ingredients:

1 Apple

5 Tsp. Honey

Step Two: Cut apple in half, remove the core, and grate your apple into a bowl.

Step Two: Add 5 teaspoons of honey and mix solution well.

Step Three: Smooth solution over skin and let sit for 20 minutes. Rinse with cool water.

Apple Sour Cream Facial

Ingredients:

½ an Apple

1 Tbsp. Sour Cream

Step One: Cut the apple in half, remove the core, and grate in a bowl.

Step Two: Add one tablespoon of sour cream and mix into a paste.

Step Three: Apply solution to your face, let sit for 25 minutes, and rinse with warm water.

Apple Olive Oil Night Cream

Ingredients:

1 Apple

1 cup of Olive Oil

1 cup of Rose Water

Step One: Cut the apple in half, remove the core, and dice the apple into small pieces.

Step Two: Place the chopped apple into the blender, turn on low, and slowly add Olive Oil and blend until it becomes a paste.

Step Three: Place a pan on the stove, fill it about a quarter of the way up with water and turn on low. Pour the mixture into a bowl and put on the pan. Heat until warm, with continuous mixing.

Step Four: Once warm, take off the stove and let cool. Add rose water and mix well.

Step Five: Apply mixture on your skin before you go to bed and keep stored in the refrigerator for 4 to 6 days.

Avocado Egg White Mask 1

Ingredients:

½ Avocados

½ Lemons

Egg White

Make-up Brush

Step One: Remove the skin from the Avocado and place the meat in a bowl.

Step Two: Squeeze in the lemon juice of half a lemon and mix the two ingredients before adding the egg white. After mixing the mixture well, add the egg white. Keep mixing until everything is mixed together.

Step Three: Put the solution on your face with the make-up brush, avoiding the eyes and mouth.

Step Four: Let this set for 10 minutes and remove from your face with cold water.

Note: Lemon juice is great for tightening up your pores. Avocado is full of healthy fats that helps moisturize the skin.

Avocado Olive Oil Mask 2

Ingredients:

½ Avocados

1 Tbsp. Olive Oil

1 Tbsp. Plain Yogurt

Step One: Take ½ an avocado and put it into a bowl. Pour in one tablespoon of Olive Oil and add one tablespoon of yogurt.

Step Two: Mash all ingredients together and mix until well incorporated.

Step Three: Apply mixture to your face and leave on face for 15 minutes. Rinse off with lukewarm water

Avocado Honey Mask 3

Ingredients:

½ an Avocado

2 Tsp. Honey

½ cup of Plain Yogurt

15 Baby Carrots

Step One: Boil the baby carrots in water until they are soft. Place the carrots in a bowl and mash with a fork.

Step Two: Add the Avocado, honey, and yogurt, and mix into a paste.

Step Three: Apply solution onto your face, nose, and neck. Let sit for 25 minutes and remove with cold water.

Avocado Coconut Hair Conditioner

1 Avocado

1 cup of Coconut Milk

Tbsp. Honey

Step One: Peel and remove seed from the avocado and place in blender. Add a little water and blend into a paste.

Step Two: Pour the avocado into a bowl, add the coconut milk and honey and mix well.

Step Three: Wash and dry your hair and apply the conditioner to your hair. Put on a shower cap and let sit for 30 minutes. After 30 minutes, remove conditioner form your hair with warm water.

Banana Cucumber Facial 1

Ingredients:

½ Bananas

2 slices of Cucumber

1 Tbsp. Honey

¼ cup Rice

¼ cup milk

Step One: Mash up the banana in a bowl. Add the honey, rice, and milk, and mix into a paste.

Step Two: Wash your hand and face with warm water and blot dry with a paper towel.

Step Three: Place a towel over your pillow, put on some soft music, apply mixture to your face, lay down and put the cucumber slices over your eyes.

Step Four: Leave the solution on for 25 minutes and rinse with cool water.

Banana Oatmeal Facial

Ingredient:

¼ cup Oatmeal

¼ cup Yogurt

½ Bananas

¼ cup Orange Juice

Popsicle Stick

Step One: Mash up the banana in a bowl and add the Oatmeal, Yogurt, and Orange Juice, and mix into a paste.

Step Two: Wash your hands and face in warm water and blot dry with a clean towel.

Step Three: Apply mixture to your face and leave on for 15 minutes.

Step Four: Remove the chunks with the Popsicle stick and rinse with warm water.

Step Five: Wet a towel in warm water and place it on your face until it cools.

Banana Honey Facial

Ingredient:

1 Banana

1 Tbsp. Honey

½ a Lemon

Step One: Mash a whole banana in a bowl with a fork. Add the honey and the juice from half a lemon.

Step Two: Mix the solution into a mix.

Step Three: Wash your hands with warm water and wash and blot dry your face. Apply the mixture with your hands as evenly as possible on your face, nose, chin, and neck.

Step Four: Let sit on your face for 10 minutes. After ten minutes, use a hot, steamy towel to pat your face clean.

Brown Sugar Olive Oil Scrub

Ingredients:

1 Tbsp. Olive oil

2 Tbsp. Brown Sugar

Step One: Pour the brown sugar in a bowl, mash up the chunks with the back of a fork. Apply the olive oil and mix to the consistency of a paste.

Step Two: Wash your hands with soap and warm water, and rinse your face with cool water and blot dry. Message the scrub into your skin using your hands in a circular motion.

Step Three: Let sit for 10 minutes rinse with warm water.

Brown Sugar Facial Scrub 2

Ingredient:

1 Tbsp. Milk

1 Tbsp. Brown Sugar

1 Tbsp. Honey

Step One: Pour all items in a bowl and mix to a paste texture.

Step Two: Apply the solution to your face with your finger tips and message into your face in a circular motion.

Step Three: Let the mixture sit on your skin for 15 minutes. Remove the solution with a small hand towel and warm water.

Cucumber Mask

Ingredients:

1 Cucumber

Blender

Step One: Peel the skin off the cucumber and cut into small pieces.

Step Two: Pour the pieces into your blender and mix on high until it becomes a paste.

Step Three: Squeeze out all the juice with a strainer and apply the paste to your face. Leave on for 15 minutes and rinse with warm water.

Cucumber Lemon Mask

Ingredients:

1 Cucumber

½ a Lemon

1 Tbsp. Witch hazel

I Egg White

Blender

Step One: Cut the cucumber into 2 inch sections, removing the skin and seeds.

Step Two: Place everything into the blender, starting with the cucumber, one egg white, witch hazel, and the juice of half a lemon.

Step Three: Use a cotton ball to apply the solution; let sit for about 15 minutes.

Step Four: Remove with a hand towel and warm water.

Cucumber Yogurt Mask

Ingredients:

1 Cucumber

½ cup of Plain Yogurt

1 Tsp. non-fat Milk Powder

Blender

Step One: Peel and remove seed from the cucumber cut into small cubes.

Step Two: Place cucumber pieces into the blender and blend to a paste. Add yogurt and powder milk and mix well.

Step Three: Apply solution on your face. Let sit for 20 minutes and rinse with warm water.

Lemon Honey Facial

Ingredients:

1 Tsp. Honey

½ a Lemon

1 drop Sweet Almond Oil

Step One: This is an anti-wrinkle mask. Mix honey, the juice of half a lemon, and a drop of sweet almond oil in a bowl.

Step Two: Apply mixture to your face with your fingertips in a circular motion and let sit for 20 minutes.

Step Three: Wash dry with warm water.

Lemon Banana Facial

Ingredients:

½ a Banana

½ a Lemon

1 Tsp. Honey

Step One: Place the banana in a bowl and mash using the back of the fork. Add one teaspoon of honey and the juice of half a lemon, mix well into a paste.

Step Two: Apply mixture to your skin and let sit for 10 minutes.

Step Three: Rinse with warm water and blot dry with towel.

Lemon Egg White Facial

1 Egg White

½ a Lemon

Large Bowl

Step One: Squeeze the lemon juice into a small bowl. Crack the egg, separate the yolk from the white, and put the white in the bowl.

Step Two: Mix the white and lemon juice together with a fork.

Step Three: Pour steaming hot water in the large bowl. Cover you head with a towel and hold your face over the steam for 5 minutes. The towel helps capture the stream.

Step Four: After 5 minutes, message the egg and lemon solution on your face. Let sit for 10 minutes, and rinse with warm water and blot dry.

Lemon Skin Toner

Ingredients:

2 Tbsp. Rubbing Alcohol

1 Tsp. Witch hazel

1 Tbsp. Distilled Water

2 Tbsp. Lemon Juice

Step One: Wash your hands and face with warm water and blot dry.

Step Two: Pour solution in a bowl and mix.

Step Three: Apply solution to your skin with a cotton ball and rinse with cool water. Store what's left in the refrigerator. It is good for up to a week.

Watermelon Skin Toner

Ingredients:

2 Tbsp. Watermelon Juice

1 Tbsp. Rubbing Alcohol

2 Tbsp. Distilled Water

Step One: Cut the watermelon in to chunks, place in a blender and blend into a liquid.

Step Two: Pour two tablespoon in a bowl and add rubbing alcohol and distilled water and mix well.

Step Three: Dip cotton ball into the solution and apply on your face let set for 10 minutes and rinse with warm water.

Tomato Skin Toner

Ingredients:

1 Tomato

¼ of a Cucumber

4 drops of Lime Juice

Cotton Ball

Step One: Wash the tomato in cold water and cut into chunks.

Step Two: Place the tomato into a blender, along with the cucumber and lime juice, and blend for 30 seconds.

Step Three: Pour solution into a bowl, dip with a cotton ball, and apply to your face and neck. Let sit for 15 minutes and rinse with warm water.

Rice Skin Toner

Ingredient:

½ cup of Rice

1 cup of Water

Step One: Rinse the rice with cold water and remove the dirt.

Step Two: Pour the rice into a bowl and fill the bowl with one cup of cold water and mix well. Soak the rice water overnight in the refrigerator.

Step Three: The next day, drain the water into a bowl. The water should have taken on a milky appearance. Apply the solution onto your face. Let sit for 20 minutes and rinse with warm water.

.

Rose Water Skin Toner

Ingredients:

¼ cup of Rosewater

Cotton Balls

Bowl

Step One: Pour ¼ cup of rosewater into a bowl.

Step Two: Wash your hands face and neck in warm soapy water and blot dry with a hand towel.

Step Three: Dip the cotton ball in the rose water and rub on your face and neck. Let sit for 20 minutes and rinse with warm water.

Witch Hazel Skin Toner

¼ cup of Witch Hazel

Cotton Ball

Step One: Pour ¼ cup of Witch Hazel into a bowl.

Step Two: Wash your hands, face, and neck with warm water and blot dry with a towel.

Step Three: Dip the cotton ball into the witch hazel and apply it to your face, nose, and neck. Use caution around the eyes. Leave on for 20 minutes and rinse with warm water.

Green Tea Skin Toner

Ingredients:

2 Tsp. Powdered Green Tea

½ cup of Boiling Water

Step One: Place green tea into boiling water for 10 minutes.

Step Two: After 10 minutes, remove from stove and let sit until cool.

Step Three: Once it's cooled down, apply solution on your face and neck with a cotton ball. Leave it on for 30 minutes and rinse with warm water. This toner is great for oily skin and safe to use daily.

Lemon Oil Skin Toner

Ingredients:

1 Teaspoon Lemon Oil

1 Teaspoon Tea Tree Oil

1 Tbsp. of Apple Cider Vinegar

½ cup water

Step One: Pour all ingredients into a bowl and mix well.

Step Two: Apply solution onto your skin with a paper towel. Let sit for 20 minutes and rinse with cold water.

This toner is great for oily skin and safe to use daily.

Tea Tree Oil Skin Toner

1 Tbsp. Tea Tree Oil

½ cup of Witch Hazel

½ Cup of Water

Step One: Pour the ingredients in a small spray bottle and shake well.

Step Two: Cover your eyes and spray the solution on your face and neck and let sit for 25 minutes.

Step Three: After 25 minutes, rinse with warm water and dry.

Rubbing Alcohol Skin Toner

Ingredients:

1 Peppermint Tea Bag

1 Tbsp. Lime Juice

¼ cup Witch Hazel

Step One: Place one cup of water in a small sauce pan and bring to a boil on the stove.

Step Two: Place the tea bag in the water and steep for 10 minutes. Remove the tea bag and let cool.

Step Three: Mix in lime juice and witch hazel and store in a bowl in the refrigerator. Apply mix to your skin and let sit for 20 minutes. Rinse with warm water.

Peppermint Tea Skin Toner

Ingredients:

1 Tbsp. Chopped Parsley

1 Tbsp. Lime Juice

¼ cup Plain Yogurt

1 Tsp. Olive Oil

2 Tbsp. Cream of Wheat

Step One: Pour plain yogurt into a bowl and add parsley, lime juice, Olive oil, and cream of wheat. Mix all ingredients into a paste.

Step Two: Apply solution onto your skin and allow it to sit for 10 minutes. After 10 minutes, rinse off with warm water.

Parsley Yogurt Skin Toner

Ingredients:

1 Tbsp. Chopped Parsley

1 Tbsp. Lime Juice

¼ cup Plain Yogurt

1 Tsp. Olive Oil

2 Tbsp. Cream of Wheat

Step One: Pour plain yogurt into a bowl add parsley, lime juice, Olive oil; and cream of wheat. Mix all mixtures into a paste.

Step Two: Apply solution onto your skin and allow it to sit for 10 minutes. After 10 minutes rinse off with warm water.

Egg White Yogurt Hair Conditioner

Ingredient:

2 Eggs

6 Tbsp. Plain Yogurt

Step One: Crack two eggs and separate the white from yolk and pour the white in a bowl.

Step Two: Add six tablespoons of yogurt and mix until it's nice and smooth.

Step Three: Massage the solution into your hair, being sure to start at the roots and work to the end of your hair.

Step Four: Cover your hair with a shower cap, leave the conditioner on for 25 minutes, and remove with shampoo and warm water.

Honey Coconut Hair Conditioner

Ingredients:

3 Tbsp. Honey

¼ cup of Coconut Oil

Step One: Pour the honey and coconut oil in a bowl mix the solution together.

Step Two: Apply mixture to your hair thoroughly. Cover your hair with a shower cap and leave on for at least 30 minutes.

Step Three: After 30 minutes, rinse off solution with warm water and shampoo.

Honey Olive Oil Hair Conditioner

2 Tbsp. Honey

2 Tbsp. Olive Oil

Step One: Pour olive oil in a bowl add honey and mix until ingredient combine.

Step Two: Apply conditioner on your hair thoroughly starting at the roots. Once applied, cover your hair with a shower cap, and leave the conditioner on for 45 minutes.

Step Three: After 45 minutes, shampoo off solution with a mild shampoo and luke warm water.

Honey Mayo Hair Conditioner

Ingredients:

1 Tbsp. Honey

1 Tbsp. Mayo

1 Egg White

Step One: Pour one tablespoon honey, one tablespoon mayo, and mix together in a bowl.

Step Two: Crack the egg, separate the white from the yolk, and pour the white in the bowl and mix.

Step Three: Apply mixture to your hair, cover with shower cap, and after 15 minutes, rinse with warm water.

Coconut Milk Banana Hair Conditioner

Ingredients:

1 Banana

1 Cup Aloe Vera Juice

½ Can Coconut Milk

¼ Cup Olive Oil

Step One: Place the banana, one cup of Aloe Vera Juice, and Olive Oil into the blender mix for 45 seconds.

Step Two: Using a strainer, pour the solution into a bowl, separating the liquid from the chunks. Using the liquid, add the coconut milk and mix well.

Step Three: Apply mixture to your hair, starting at the roots and working toward the ends of your hair.

Step Four: Cover your hair with a shower cap and leave solution on 30 minutes. Shampoo your hair with a mild shampoo and rinse hair with warm water.

Avocado Banana Hair Conditioner

Ingredients:

½ Avocado

1 Banana

1 Tbsp. Olive Oil

Step One: Remove the skin and seed from avocado and place in a bowl. Add banana.

Step Two: Mash items into a paste using a fork. Add olive oil and mix well.

Step Three: Apply solution to your hair, starting at the root of your hair and work to the ends. Cover your hair with a shower cap for 30 minutes. Rinse with warm water.

Thank you so much for taking the time to read this book. I hope your skin care regimen is an easy and simple process.

Now I'd like ask for a *small* favor. If you found this book to be useful, please take a few minutes to leave a review on Amazon...

...Even a few sentences will help!

Here's the link again:

amazon.com/author/marciasavage e

This feedback will help me to write the kind of Kindle books that help you get results. And if you loved it, please let me know.

Order Books by Ann Savage:

18 Beauty Recipes

Greatest Beauty Secrets of All Time!

http://www.amazon.com/dp/B00KKO6CQC

More Kindle eBooks By Marcia Savage:

CLEAN HOUSE IN 30 MINUTES

http://www.amazon.com/CLEAN-HOUSE-IN-30-MINUTES-ebook/dp/B00HVS4TZG

AN ORGANIZED HOME IN 30 MINUTES

http://www.amazon.com/AN-ORGANIZED-HOME-IN-MINUTES-ebook/dp/B00IGKZU0G

BEST HOMEMADE STAIN REMOVER EVER

http://www.amazon.com/BEST-HOMEMADE-STAIN-REMOVER-EVER-ebook/dp/B00IPQ1VF4

28 NATURAL HAIR REMEDIES TO MAKE YOUR HAIR GROWTH FASTER

http://www.amazon.com/dp/B00KFUTZ8S

29 EASY STEPS TO SPEED CLEAN YOUR HOUSE

http://www.amazon.com/dp/B00KET50T8

88 EASY STEPS TO SIMPLIFY YOUR HOUSE CLEANING

http://www.amazon.com/dp/B00KAG2NMC

35 Easy Ways To Get Rid Of Acne Fast

http://www.amazon.com/dp/B00JWF1LA2

20 CREATIVE WAYS TO REMOVE STAINS USING MOTHER'S GREEN CLEANING PRODUCTS

http://www.amazon.com/dp/B00JZ5O45S